The Fastest Keto Muffins and Creams Recipes

The Best Muffins and Ice Creams Recipes to Enjoy while doing Keto and Lose Weight Easier

Jessica Simpson

1

Contents

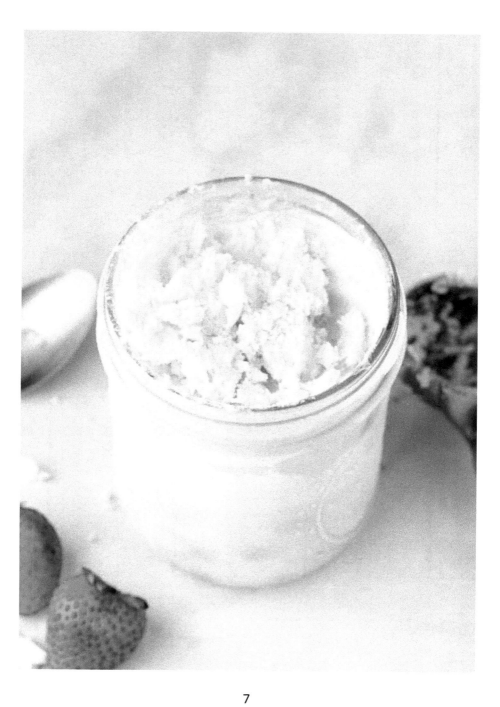

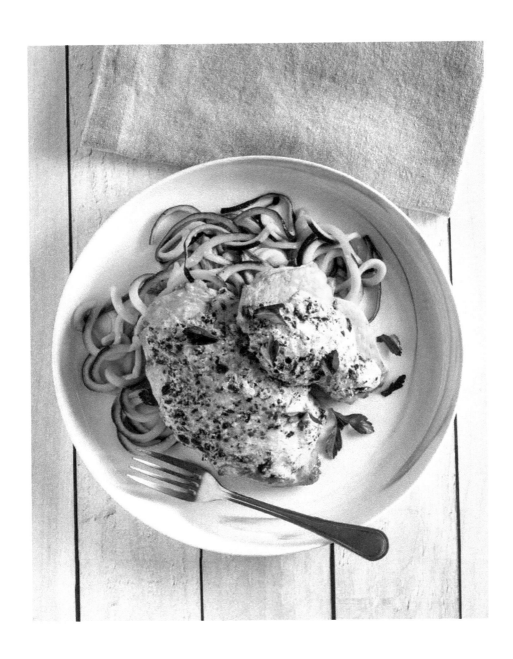

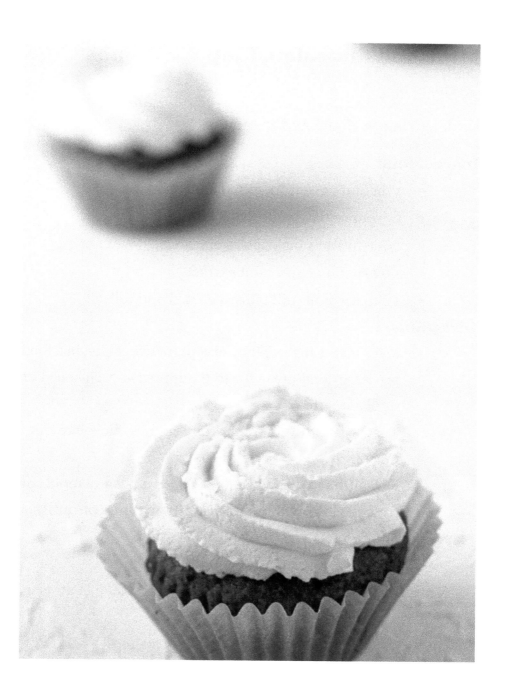

Mint And Chocolate Chip Ice Bombs

Servings: 14

Cooking Time: 3 Hours And 10 Minutes

Ingredients:

- 1 medium avocado, pitted and peeled
- 2.1-ounce dark chocolate, chopped
- 1/4 cup and 1 tablespoon erythritol sweetener
- 1 teaspoon peppermint extract
- 1 cup coconut milk, unsweetened and full-fat

Directions:

1. Place all the ingredients, except for chocolate, in a food processor and pulse for to 2 minutes at high speed or until smooth.
2. Tip the mixture in a bowl and fold in chocolate until mixed.
3. Divide the mixture evenly between 14 candy molds or round cake mold and freeze for 2 to hours or until set and firm.
4. Serve when ready.

Nutrition Info: Calories: 67 Cal, Carbs: 2.8 g, Fat: 6 g, Protein: 0.g, Fiber: 1.1 g.

Blueberry Lemon Cheesecake

Servings: 6

Cooking Time: 0 Minute

Ingredients:

- 8 oz cream cheese
- 1/2 cup heavy whipping cream
- 1/4 cup sour cream
- 1/2 cup swerve confectioner
- 3 ounces blueberries
- 1 tsp vanilla essence
- 15 drops liquid stevia
- 1 lemon zest
- 1 lemon juice
- 6 popsicle silicone molds

Directions:

1. Beat the sour cream with heavy cream in a mixer.
2. Whisk in lemon zest, juice, stevia, swerve and vanilla essence.
3. Add berries and mix well while mashing the berries with a spoon.
4. Pour this mixture into suitable popsicle molds and insert ice cream sticks in it.
5. Freeze them for 6 hours or more.
6. Remove the popsicles from the molds.

7. Serve.

Nutrition Info: Per Servings: Calories 213 Total Fat 19 g Saturated Fat 15.2 g Cholesterol 13 mg Total Carbs 5.5 g Sugar 1.3 g Fiber 0.5 g Sodium 52 mg Potassium mg Protein 6.1 g

Lemon And Raspberry Sorbet

Servings: 6

Cooking Time:10 Minutes

Ingredients:

- 3 cups frozen raspberries
- Juice of 3 ripe lemons
- 1 tsp Stevia/your preferred keto sweetener
- 3 Tbsp coconut oil

Directions:

1. Place all ingredients into a food processor and blend until completely smooth
2. Transfer the sorbet into an ice cream container or plastic container and smooth out the top
3. Place the lid on top and place the sorbet into the freezer. Give it a good stir every hour for the first five hours to help the texture to become creamy as opposed to icy
4. Serve with a lemon wedge and enjoy!

Nutrition Info: Calories: 97;Fat: 7 grams ;Protein: 1 gram ;Total carbs: 9 grams;Net carbs: grams

Mix Berry Popsicles

Servings: 4

Cooking Time: 0 Minute

Ingredients:

- 5 oz cream cheese
- 1/4 cup full-fat coconut milk
- 3 tbsp yogurt
- 1/4 cup powdered erythritol
- 2 tbsp shredded coconut
- 1 tsp chia seeds
- 1/4 cup frozen strawberries
- 1/4 cup frozen blueberries
- 1/4 cup frozen blackberries
- 1/2 tsp MCT oil

Directions:

1. First blend all the popsicle ingredients in a blender except the berries.
2. Now add berries and pulse for seconds to break the berries into pieces.
3. Pour this mixture into suitable popsicle molds and insert ice cream sticks in it.
4. Freeze them for 2 hours or more.
5. Remove the popsicles from the molds.
6. Serve.

Nutrition Info: Per Servings: Calories 19Total Fat 19.2 g Saturated Fat 10.1 g Cholesterol 11 mg Total Carbs 7.3 g Sugar 1.2 g Fiber 0.8 g Sodium 78 mg Potassium 109 mg Protein 4.2 g

Creamy Raspberry Cheesecake Ice Cream

Servings: 8

Cooking Time: 30 Minutes

Ingredients:

- 1 tbsp swerve
- 4 oz raspberries
- 1 tsp vanilla
- ½ cup unsweetened almond milk
- 1 ½ cups heavy cream
- ¾ cup Swerve
- 8 oz cream cheese, softened

Directions:

1. In a large bowl, beat together cream cheese and swerve until smooth.
2. Add vanilla, almond milk, and heavy cream and mix well.
3. Pour ice cream mixture into the ice cream maker and churn according to machine instructions.
4. In a small bowl, mash raspberries. Add 1 tbsp swerve in mashed raspberries and mix well.
5. Add mash raspberry mixture to the ice cream.
6. Serve and enjoy.

Nutrition Info: Per Servings: Net Carbs: 2.5g; Calories: 188 Total Fat: 18.5g; Saturated Fat: 11.4g Protein: 2.8g; Carbs: 3.5g; Fiber: 1g; Sugar: 0.8g; Fat 89% Protein 6% Carbs 5%

Coffee Cheesecake Ice Cream

Servings: 8

Cooking Time:15 Minutes

Ingredients:

- 2 cups heavy cream
- 1 ½ tsp Stevia/your preferred keto sweetener
- 4 tsp instant espresso powder
- 9 oz plain, full-fat cream cheese

Directions:

1. Whip the cream, stevia and instant coffee powder until soft, fluffy and thick, set aside
2. Give the cream cheese a good, hard stir to soften it
3. Fold the whipped cream mixture into the stirred cream cheese until combined
4. Spoon the mixture into an ice cream container or plastic container, place the lid on top and pop it into the freezer
5. Give the ice cream a good stir every hour for the first five hours of freezing time. This will help to achieve a fluffy, creamy texture
6. Serve alone, with coffee or as an accompaniment to keto cake or brownie!

Nutrition Info: Calories: 281 ;Fat: 29 grams ;Protein: 3 grams ;Total carbs: 3 grams ;Net carbs: 3 grams

Raspberry Ice Cream

Servings: 3

Cooking Time: 0 Minutes

Ingredients:

- 2 cups frozen raspberries unsweetened
- 1 cup full-fat Greek yogurt
- Powdered Swerve, to taste

Directions:

1. Beat everything in a food processor until smooth.
2. Transfer the yogurt mixture to a sealable bowl.
3. Place the mixture in the freezer for about 4 hours.
4. During this time, churn this ice cream in an ice cream maker after every 30 minutes.
5. Serve.

Nutrition Info: Calories 101 ;Total Fat 15.5 g ;Saturated Fat 4.5 g ;Cholesterol 12 mg ;Sodium 18 mg ;Total Carbs 4.4 g ;Sugar 1.2 g ;Fiber 0.3 g ;Protein 4.8 g

Yogurt

Servings: 12

Cooking Time: 1 Hour

Ingredients:

- 1 tsp. vanilla extract, sugar-free
- 8 oz. mango, diced
- 1 cup Greek yogurt
- 8 oz. strawberries, diced
- 1/2 cup heavy whipping cream

Directions:

1. In a food processor set on high, whip the yogurt until fluffy.
2. Blend the strawberries, vanilla extract, mango and heavy whipping cream until smooth.
3. Transfer to popsicle molds and freeze for 2 hours.
4. Tricks and Tips:
5. This recipe will also make soft serve ice cream that can be served after mixing the ingredients. There is no need to freeze.

Nutrition Info: 1 gram ;Net Carbs: 5 grams ;Fat: grams ;Calories: 80

Chocolate Zucchini Muffins

Servings: 9

Cooking Time: 30 Minutes

Ingredients:

- ½ cup coconut flour
- ¾ tsp baking soda
- 2 tbsp cocoa powder
- ½ tsp salt
- 1 tsp cinnamon
- ½ tsp nutmeg
- 3 large eggs
- 2/3 cup Swerve sweetener
- 2 tsp vanilla extract
- 1 tbsp oil
- 1 medium zucchini, grated
- ¼ cup heavy cream
- 1/3 cup Lily's chocolate baking chips

Directions:

1. Preheat your oven at 356 degrees F.
2. Layer a 9-cup 0 muffin tray with muffin liners then spray them with cooking oil.
3. Whisk coconut flour with salt, cinnamon, nutmeg, sweetener, baking soda, and cocoa powder in a bowl.

4. Beat eggs in a separate bowl then add oil, cream, vanilla, and zucchini.
5. Stir in the coconut flour mixture and mix well until fully incorporated.
6. Fold in chocolate chips then divide the batter into the lined muffin cups.
7. Bake these muffins for 30 minutes then allow them to cool on a wire rack.
8. Enjoy.

Nutrition Info: Calories 151 Total Fat 14.7 g Saturated Fat 1.5 g Cholesterol 13 mg Sodium 53 mg Total Carbs 1.5 g Sugar 0.3 g Fiber 0.1 g Protein 0.8 g

Buns With Psyllium Husk

Servings: 5

Cooking Time: 30 Minutes

Ingredients:

- 4 tbsp boiling water
- Dry Ingredients
- 3.53 oz blanched almond flour
- 2 tbsp psyllium husk powder
- 1 tsp baking powder
- 1 tsp black sesame seeds
- 1 tsp white sesame seeds
- 2 tsp sunflower seeds
- 1 tsp black chia seeds
- ½ tsp Himalayan salt
- ½ tsp garlic powder
- Wet Ingredients
- 1 egg
- 2 egg whites
- 1 tbsp apple cider vinegar
- 3 tbsp melted refined coconut oil

Directions:

1. Preheat your oven at 356 degrees F.
2. Add dry ingredients to a bowl along with wet ingredients. Mix well until smooth.

3. Slowly add boiled water into the dough and mix well to absorb the water.

4. Divide the dough into 5 balls, grease them with cooking oil.and roll them in your hands.

5. Place the balls on a baking sheet lined with parchment paper.

6. Bake them for 30 minutes until golden.

7. Enjoy.

Nutrition Info: Calories 76 Total Fat 7.2 g Saturated Fat 6.4 g Cholesterol 134 mg Sodium mg Total Carbs 2g Sugar 1 g Fiber 0.7 g Protein 2.2 g

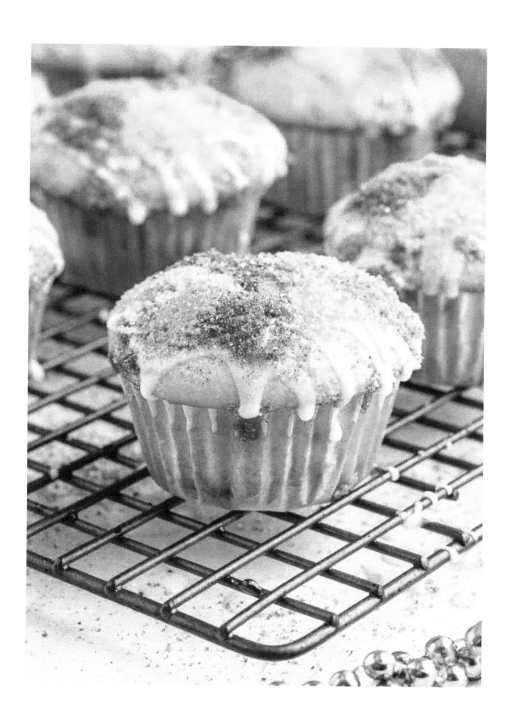

Cinnamon Roll Muffins

Servings: 6

Cooking Time: 15 Minutes

Ingredients:

- ½ cup almond flour
- 2 scoops vanilla protein powder
- 1 tsp baking powder
- 1 tbsp cinnamon
- ½ cup almond butter
- ½ cup pumpkin puree
- ½ cup coconut oil
- For the Glaze
- ¼ cup coconut butter
- ¼ cup milk of choice
- 1 tbsp granulated sweetener
- 2 tsp lemon juice

Directions:

1. Let your oven preheat at 350 degrees F. Layer a -cup muffin tray with muffin liners.
2. Add all the dry ingredients to a suitable mixing bowl then whisk in all the wet ingredients.
3. Mix until well combined then divide the batter into the muffin cups.

4. Bake them for 15 minutes then allow the muffins to cool on a wire rack.
5. Prepare the cinnamon glaze in a small bowl then drizzle this glaze over the muffins.
6. Enjoy.

Nutrition Info: Calories 252 Total Fat 13 g Saturated Fat 11.5 g Cholesterol 141 mg Sodium 153 mg Total Carbs 7.2 g Sugar 0.3 g Fiber 1.4 g Protein 5.2 g

Fathead Rolls

Servings: 6

Cooking Time: 12 Minutes

Ingredients:

- 2 oz cream cheese
- ¾ cup shredded mozzarella
- 1 egg beaten
- ¼ tsp garlic powder
- 1/3 cup almond flour
- 2 tsp baking powder
- ½ cup shredded cheddar cheese

Directions:

1. Preheat your oven at 425 degrees F.
2. Heat mozzarella and cream cheese in a small bowl for seconds in the microwave.
3. Beat egg with all the dry ingredients in a separate bowl.
4. Stir in cheese mixture to make a sticky dough adding the cheddar cheese at the end.
5. Mix well then wrap the dough in plastic wrap.
6. Refrigerate this dough for 30 minutes then divide it into 4 equal parts.
7. Cut each ball in half and place them flat side down on a baking sheet lined with wax paper.

8. Bake them for 12 minutes until golden.

9. Enjoy.

Nutrition Info: Calories 193 Total Fat g Saturated Fat 13.2 g Cholesterol 120 mg Sodium 8 mg Total Carbs 2.5 g Sugar 1 g Fiber 0.7 g Protein 2.2 g

Banana Muffins

Servings: 12

Cooking Time: 18 Minutes

Ingredients:

- 3 large eggs
- 2 cups bananas, mashed (3-4 medium bananas)
- ½ cup almond butter (peanut butter can also be used)
- ¼ cup butter (olive oil can also be used)
- 1 tsp vanilla
- ½ cup coconut flour (almond flour can also be used)
- 1 tbsp cinnamon
- 1 tsp baking powder
- 1 tsp baking soda
- Pinch sea salt
- ½ cup chocolate chips

Directions:

1. Preheat your oven at 356 degrees F.
2. Line a 1cup muffin tray with paper liners.
3. Whisk eggs with almond butter, vanilla, butter, and mashed bananas in a large bowl.
4. Stir in coconut flour, baking soda, cinnamon, baking powder, and salt. Mix well with a wooden spoon.
5. Divide this batter into the muffin cups then bake them for 18 minutes.

6. Allow them to cool then refrigerate for 30 minutes.

7. Enjoy.

Nutrition Info: Calories 139 Total Fat 4.6 g Saturated Fat 0.5 g Cholesterol 1.2 mg Sodium mg Total Carbs 7.5 g Sugar 6.3 g Fiber 0.6 g Protein 3.8 g

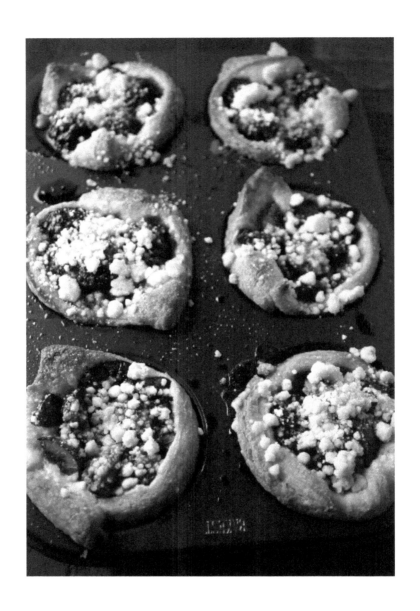

Blackberry-filled Lemon Muffins

Servings: 12

Cooking Time: 30 Minutes

Ingredients:

- For the Blackberry Filling:
- 3 tbsp granulated stevia
- 1 tsp lemon juice
- ¼ tsp xanthan gum
- 2 tbsp water
- 1 cup fresh blackberries
- For the Muffin Batter:
- 2 ½ cups super fine almond flour
- ¾ cup granulasted stevia
- 1 tsp fresh lemon zest
- ½ tsp sea salt
- 1 tsp grain-free baking powder
- 4 large eggs
- ¼ cup unsweetened almond milk
- ¼ cup butter
- 1 tsp vanilla extract
- ½ tsp lemon extract

Directions:

1. For the Blackberry Filling:

2. Add granulated sweetener and xanthan gum in a saucepan.
3. Stir in lemon juice and water then place it over the medium heat.
4. Add blackberries and stir cook on low heat for 10 minutes.
5. Remove the saucepan from the heat and allow the mixture to cool.
6. For the Muffin Batter:
7. Preheat your oven at 356 degrees F and layer a muffin tray with paper cups.
8. Mix almond flour with salt, baking powder, lemon zest, baking powder, and sweetener in a mixing bowl.
9. Whisk in eggs, vanilla extract, lemon extract, butter, and almond milk.
10. Beat well until smooth. Divide half of this batter into the muffin tray.
11. Make a depression at the center of each muffin.
12. Add a spoonful of blackberry jam mixture to each depression.
13. Cover the filling with remaining batter on top.
14. Bake the muffins for 30 minutes then allow them to cool.
15. Refrigerate for a few hours before serving.
16. Enjoy.

Nutrition Info: Calories 261 Total Fat 7.1 g Saturated Fat 13.4 g Cholesterol 0.3 mg Sodium 10 mg Total Carbs 6.1 g Sugar 2.1 g Fiber 3.9 g Protein 1.8 g

Dinner Rolls

Servings: 8

Cooking Time: 12 Minutes

Ingredients:

- 1 cup mozzarella, shredded
- 1 oz cream cheese
- 1 cup almond flour
- ¼ cup ground flaxseed
- 1 egg
- ½ tsp baking soda

Directions:

1. Preheat your oven at 400 degrees F.
2. Layer a baking sheet with wax paper and set it aside.
3. Melt mozzarella and cream cheese in a medium bowl by heating the mixture for 1 minute in the microwave.
4. Mix well then add the egg. Whisk well until combined.
5. Add baking soda, flaxseed, and almond flour.
6. Mix well to form a smooth dough then make balls out of this dough.
7. Place the balls on the baking sheet lined with wax paper.
8. Sprinkle sesame seeds over the balls.
9. Bake them for 12 minutes until golden brown.
10. Enjoy.

Nutrition Info: Calories 136 Total Fat 10.7 g Saturated Fat 0.5 g Cholesterol 4 mg Sodium 45 mg Total Carbs 1.2 g Sugar 1.4 g Fiber 0.2 g Protein 0.9

Muffins With Blueberries

Servings: 8

Cooking Time: 25 Minutes

Ingredients:

- ¾ cup coconut flour
- 6 eggs
- ½ cup coconut oil, melted
- 1/3 cup unsweetened coconut milk
- ½ cup fresh blueberries
- 1/3 cup granulated sweetener
- 1 tsp vanilla extract
- 1 tsp baking powder

Directions:

1. Preheat your oven at 356 degrees F.
2. Mix coconut flour with all the other ingredients except blueberries in a mixing bowl until smooth.
3. Stir in blueberries and mix gently.
4. Divide this batter in a greased muffin tray evenly.
5. Bake the muffins for 2minutes until golden brown.
6. Enjoy.

Nutrition Info: Calories 195 Total Fat 14.3 g Saturated Fat 10.5 g Cholesterol 1 mg Sodium 125 mg Total Carbs 4.5 g Sugar 0.5 g Fiber 0.3 g Protein 3.2 g

Breakfast Buns

Servings: 4

Cooking Time: 25 Minutes

Ingredients:

- 3 egg whites, room temperature
- 1 egg, room temperature
- ¼ cup boiling hot water
- ¼ cup almond flour
- ¼ cup coconut flour
- 1 tbsp psyllium husk powder
- 1 tsp baking powder
- Sesame seeds, for sprinkling

Directions:

1. Preheat your oven at 356 degrees F.
2. Add everything to a food processor and blend for seconds until smooth.
3. Let it sit for 20 minutes then divide the dough into 4 equal parts.
4. Shape the dough into buns then place them on a baking sheet lined with wax paper.
5. Score the top of each bun with a fork and sprinkle sesame seeds on top.
6. Bake the buns for 25 minutes until golden brown.
7. Enjoy.

Nutrition Info: Calories 200 Total Fat 11.1 g Saturated Fat 9.5 g Cholesterol 124.2 mg Sodium 46 mg Total Carbs 1.1 g Sugar 1.3 g Fiber 0.4 g Protein 0.4 g

Keto Blueberry Pie

Servings: 8

Cooking Time: 25 Minutes

Ingredients:

- Crust
- 1/2 tablespoon water
- ½ cup butter, unsalted and melted
- 2 large eggs
- ¼ teaspoon salt
- ¾ cup coconut flour
- 1/8 teaspoon baking powder
- Filling
- 1 tablespoons swerve
- 3/4 cup blueberries
- 8-ounce cream cheese

Directions:

1. Crust Instructions
2. Prepare the crust dough by mixing all of the crust ingredients.
3. Divide this dough into two equal halves.
4. Roll both the halves into two-6-inch round sheets.
5. Place one sheet in a greased 6-inch pie plate and set the pan aside.
6. Pie Instructions

7. Let your oven preheat at 350 degrees F.

8. Spread cream cheese over the base layer of the crust.

9. Mix blueberries with 2 tbsp sweeteners in a bowl.

10. Spread this berry mixture over the cream cheese layer.

11. Place the other sheet of the dough on top of the filling.

12. Press and pinch the dough around the edges to seal the pie.

13. Bake the pie for 25 minutes in the preheated oven.

14. Allow the baked pie to cool at room temperature.

15. Slice and serve.

Nutrition Info: Per Servings: Calories 236 Total Fat 21.5 g Saturated Fat 15.2 g Cholesterol 54 mg Total Carbs 7.6 g Sugar 1.4 g Fiber 3.8 g Sodium 21 mg Potassium 41 mg Protein 4.3 g

Low Carb Samoa Pie

Servings: 8

Cooking Time: 0 Minute

Ingredients:

- Chocolate Crust
- 1/2 cup sunflower seeds raw, unsalted
- 1/2 cup sugar free cocoa powder
- 1/2 cup coconut flour
- 1/2 cup Swerve
- 1/2 tsp salt
- 8 tbsp butter soft
- Filling
- 16 ounces heavy whipping cream
- 1 tsp vanilla liquid stevia
- 8 ounces cream cheese softened
- Topping
- 1/2 cup Coconut flakes sugar free, toasted
- 2 ounces my Microwave Salted Caramel Sauce
- 2 ounces Sugar-Free Chocolate Chips
- 3 tsp butter

Directions:

1. Add and blend all the ingredients for the crust in a food processor.

2. Pulse the processor to blend everything together until smooth.

3. Spread this mixture into 9-inch pie pan and press it down. Set it aside.

4. Beat heavy cream with stevia and vanilla in a bowl.

5. Whisk the cream cheese in an electric mixer and stir in cream mixture.

6. Mix well then spread this filling into the pie crust.

7. Toss coconut flakes in a caramel sauce to prepare the topping.

8. Drizzle melted chocolate and caramel sauce mixture over the filling.

9. Refrigerate the pie for 3 hours.

10. Slice and serve.

Nutrition Info: Per Servings: Calories 190 Total Fat 17.25 g Saturated Fat 7.1 g Cholesterol 20 mg Total Carbs 5.5 g Sugar 2.8 g Fiber 3.8 g Sodium 28 mg Potassium 47 mg Protein 3 g

Coconut Pie

Servings: 8

Cooking Time: 20 Minutes

Ingredients:

- 2 oz shredded coconut
- 14 cup erythritol
- 14 cup coconut oil
- 5.5 oz coconut flakes
- 1 tsp xanthan gum
- 34 cup erythritol
- 2 cups heavy cream

Directions:

1. Add coconut flakes, erythritol, and coconut oil into the food processor and process for 30-40 seconds.
2. Transfer coconut flakes mixed into the pie pan and spread evenly.
3. Lightly press down the mixture and bake at 0 F 180 C for 10 minutes.
4. Heat heavy cream in a saucepan over low heat.
5. Whisk in shredded coconut, powdered erythritol, and xanthan gum. Bring to boil.
6. Remove from heat and set aside to cool for 10 minutes.
7. Pour filling mixture onto the crust and place in the refrigerator for overnight.

8. Slice and serve.

Nutrition Info: Per Servings: Net Carbs: 2.5g; Calories: 206; Total Fat: 21.4g; Saturated Fat: 15. Protein: 1.1g; Carbs: 3.8g; Fiber: 1.3g; Sugar: 1.7g; Fat 93% Protein 3% Carbs 4%

Vegan Keto Chocolate Almond Butter Pie

Servings: 24

Cooking Time: 30 Minutes

Ingredients:

- For crust:
- 1 ½ cups coconut flour
- 1 cup coconut oil, melted
- ¼ teaspoon salt
- 4 tablespoons psyllium husk
- 1 cup water
- For filling:
- 4 ounces unsweetened chocolate
- ½ cup coconut oil
- ½ teaspoon stevia (optional)
- 2 cans (14.5 ounces each) full fat coconut milk
- 2 cups almond butter

Directions:

1. To make crust: Add water and coconut oil into a bowl. Add psyllium husk and mix well. Stir for about a minute.
2. Add coconut flour and salt and stir. Let it rest for a couple of minutes. The mixture should be dry by now.
3. Divide the dough into 2 pie pans (9 inches each). Press it well onto the bottom and side of the pan.

4. Prick the crust in a few places with a fork.

5. Bake in a preheated oven at 3° F for around 30 minutes or until light golden brown on top. Remove from the oven and let it cool for 15 minutes.

6. Meanwhile, melt the chocolate in a double boiler or microwave and pour into a blender.

7. Add the rest of the ingredients for the filling and blend until smooth. Pour over the crust.

8. Refrigerate for 9 hours.

9. Slice and serve.

10. Transfer leftovers into an airtight container. Refrigerate until use. These can keep for 4 days.

Nutrition Info: Per Servings: Calories: 3kcal, Fat: 36 g, Carbohydrates: 5.5 g, Protein: 7.2 g

Butter

Servings: 24

Cooking Time: 1 Hour

Ingredients:

- For the crust:
- 1/8 tsp. salt1/4 cup sweetener, granulated
- 1 cup butter2 cups almond flour
- For the filling:
- 3 tbsp. almond flour
- 1/4 cup butter1 tbsp. baking powder, gluten-free
- 3 large eggs, beaten1 tsp. vanilla extract, sugar-free
- 1 1/4 cups Sukrin Gold brown sugar substitute
- 3/4 cup coconut, unsweetened
- 1/8 tsp. salt

Directions:

1. Set your oven to the temperature of 350° Fahrenheit. Heavily coat a x 9 baking pan with butter.
2. In a big dish, mix the sweetener and butter with an electrical beater until combined. Then blend the almond flour and salt to the mixture until soft.
3. Distribute the dough to the prepared baking pan and spread evenly. Use an additional big dish to cream the butter with an electrical beater until fluffy. Blend the

eggs, brown sugar substitute, and vanilla extract and whip until combined.

4. Add the almond flour and salt to the mixture and combine thoroughly. Fold in the coconut and baking powder with a rubber scraper until totally incorporated.

5. Pour the filling over the dough in the prepared baking pan.

6. Heat in the stove for 30 - 35 minutes.Move to cool on the counter completely before cutting into squares.

Nutrition Info: 3 grams ;Net Carbs: 6.9 grams ;Fat: 14 grams ;Calories: 1

Cherry Limeade Pops

Servings: 4-5

Cooking Time: 10 Minutes

Ingredients:

- 1 ½ cups pitted cherries
- 1 tablespoon erythritol
- Juice of a lime
- ½ cup water

Directions:

1. Add cherries, erythritol, lime juice and water into a small pan. Place the pan over medium heat. Stir frequently. Cook for 8 – minutes or until the cherries are soft. Mash the cherries with the back of the spoon, or potato masher as they cook.
2. Turn off the heat and let the mix cool to room temperature.
3. Divide into 4-5 Popsicle molds. Insert the popsicle sticks and freeze until firm.
4. To serve: Dip the Popsicle molds in a bowl of warm water for 15 – 20 seconds. The Popsicles will loosen up. Remove from the molds and serve.

Nutrition Info: per Servings: Calories: 1kcal, Fat: 0 g, Carbohydrates: 3.6 g, Protein: 0.4 g

Keto Peanut Butter Blondies

Servings: 8

Cooking Time: 15 - 18 Minutes

Ingredients:

- 2 ounces butter, melted, slightly cooled (or substitute with 3 ½ tablespoons coconut oil and ½ tablespoon coconut cream)
- 2 ounces natural peanut butter
- 1 teaspoon vanilla extract
- ½ teaspoon salt
- 1/3 cup dark chocolate chips or chunks + extra to top
- 1/3 cup powdered erythritol
- 2 eggs, at room temperature
- 2 ounces almond flour
- ¼ teaspoon + 1/8 teaspoon baking powder
- Flaky sea salt, to garnish (optional)

Directions:

1. Place rack in the lower third position in the oven. Place a sheet of parchment paper in a 6 x 6 inch baking dish.
2. Place peanut butter, butter and sweetener in a bowl and beat until well incorporated.
3. Beat in the eggs, one at a time and beat well each time.
4. Beat in the almond flour, baking powder and salt until well combined and free from lumps.

5. Add chocolate chips and fold gently. Spoon the batter into the baking dish. Scatter some chocolate chips on top if desired.
6. Bake in a preheated oven 350° F for about 20 – 22 minutes. It should be almost set but not firm, slightly undercooked. Sprinkle flaky salt on top, if using.
7. Remove from the oven and let cool on a wire rack.
8. Cut into equal squares and serve.
9. Transfer leftovers into airtight container. Refrigerate until use. These can keep for 5-6 days or up to a month in the freezer.

Nutrition Info: Per Servings: Calories: 146 kcal, Fat: 13.1 g, Carbohydrates: 4.6 g, Protein: 4 g

Baked Vanilla Cheesecake

Servings: 12

Cooking Time:2 Hours

Ingredients:

- Cookies for the base:
- 5 oz butter, softened
- 2 eggs
- 1 tsp Stevia/your preferred keto sweetener
- 1 tsp baking powder
- 1 ½ cups ground almonds
- 1 cup finely chopped walnuts
- To make the base:
- All of the cookies you baked!
- 4 oz melted butter
- Cheesecake filling:
- 1 lb plain cream cheese
- 10 ½ oz full fat sour cream
- 3 eggs
- 1 Tbsp vanilla extract
- 1 tsp Stevia/your preferred keto sweetener

Directions:

1. Bake the cookies: preheat the oven to 360 degrees Fahrenheit and line a baking tray with baking paper. Beat the butter until soft and creamy. Add the eggs to

the butter and beat thoroughly. Stir the sweetener, baking powder, ground almonds and walnuts into the egg/butter mix. Roll the dough into balls, place onto the lined tray, press down with a fork and bake for 20 minutes or until golden. Leave to cool completely

2. Preheat the oven to 360 degrees Fahrenheit and line a cake pan with baking paper and set aside

3. Place the cooked and cooled cookies into a food processor with the melted butter and pulse until you achieve a wet, sandy consistency

4. Press the cookie/butter mix into your lined cake pan and set aside

5. Pop the cream cheese and sour cream into the food processor and blitz until smooth and creamy. Add the eggs, vanilla and sweetener and process until combined and smooth

6. Pour the cream cheese mixture into your cookie-lined cake pan and pop it into the oven to bake for about an hour or until the edges of the cheesecake are cooked but the middle is still a little gooey

7. Leave to cool completely before slicing and serving!

Nutrition Info: Calories: 476;Fat: 47 grams ;Protein: 10 grams ;Total carbs: 6 grams ;Net carbs: 4 grams

Chocolate Hazelnut Tart

Servings: 12

Cooking Time:45 Minutes

Ingredients:

- 1 cup ground hazelnuts
- ⅓ cup ground almonds
- 5 oz butter, melted
- 1 tsp Stevia/your preferred keto sweetener
- 7 oz 72% cocoa dark chocolate
- 3 oz butter
- 4 egg yolks
- ¾ cup heavy cream
- 1 tsp hazelnut essence (optional)
- 2 tsp Stevia/your preferred keto sweetener
- 1 tsp sea salt
- Sea salt to sprinkle over top (optional)

Directions:

1. Preheat the oven to 360 degrees Fahrenheit and thoroughly grease a pie dish with butter
2. Combine the ground hazelnuts, ground almonds, melted butter and the first measure of sweetener until you have a sandy-textured mixture
3. Press the nut mixture into your prepared pie dish and try your best to press the mixture up the sides

4. Pop the pie dish into the oven to allow the nutty base to bake for 10 minutes

5. Make the filling: place the chocolate and butter into a heatproof bowl and place over a saucepan of boiling water. Stir as the chocolate and butter melt together. Remove from the heat and leave to cool

6. Whisk the egg yolks, cream, hazelnut essence, sweetener and sea salt into the chocolate mixture until super smooth

7. Pour the filling into the prebaked pie crust and place back into the oven to bake for about 15 minutes or until the filling is just set but still a little wobbly in the center

8. Leave the pie to cool before serving

9. Optional: sprinkle the pie with a little pinch of sea salt before serving

Nutrition Info: Calories: 400;Fat: 39 grams ;Protein: 6 grams ;Total carbs: 9 grams ;Net carbs: 4 grams

Ketogenic Cheese Cake

Servings: 6

Cooking Time: 50 Minutes

Ingredients:

- For the Almond Flour Cheesecake Crust:
- 2 Cups of Blanched almond flour
- 1/3 Cup of almond Butter
- 3 Tablespoons of Erythritol (powdered or granular)
- 1 Teaspoon of Vanilla extract
- For the Keto Cheesecake Filling:
- 32 Oz of softened Cream cheese
- 1 and ¼ cups of powdered erythritol
- 3 Large Eggs
- 1 Tablespoon of Lemon juice
- 1 Teaspoon of Vanilla extract

Directions:

1. Preheat your oven to a temperature of about 350 degrees F.
2. Grease a spring form pan of 9¨ with cooking spray or just line its bottom with a parchment paper.
3. In order to make the cheesecake rust, stir in the melted butter, the almond flour, the vanilla extract and the erythritol in a large bowl.

4. The dough will get will be a bit crumbly; so press it into the bottom of your prepared tray.
5. Bake for about 12 minutes; then let cool for about 10 minutes.
6. In the meantime, beat the softened cream cheese and the powdered sweetener at a low speed until it becomes smooth.
7. Crack in the eggs and beat them in at a low to medium speed until it becomes fluffy. Make sure to add one a time.
8. Add in the lemon juice and the vanilla extract and mix at a low to medium speed with a mixer.
9. Pour your filling into your pan right on top of the crust. You can use a spatula to smooth the top of the cake.
10. Bake for about 45 to 50 minutes.
11. Remove the baked cheesecake from your oven and run a knife around its edge.
12. Let the cake cool for about 4 hours in the refrigerator.
13. Serve and enjoy your delicious cheese cake!

Nutrition Info: Calories: 325;Fat: 29g;Carbohydrates: 6g;Fiber: 1g;Protein: 7g

Fudgy Cocoa Brownies (paleo And Keto)

Servings: 8

Cooking Time: 18-20 Minutes

Ingredients:

- 2 ounces unsalted butter for keto or 4 tablespoons coconut oil + ½ tablespoon coconut cream for Paleo
- 1.5 ounces cocoa powder, unsweetened
- 1 egg, at room temperature
- ½ cup erythritol for keto or coconut sugar for Paleo or add more to taste
- ¼ teaspoon salt
- 1 ounce almond flour
- To serve:
- Flaky sea salt
- Unsweetened, cold macadamia milk

Directions:

1. Place rack in the lower third position in the oven. Place a sheet of parchment paper in a 6 x 6 inch baking dish.
2. Add butter, cocoa, sweetener and salt into a heatproof bowl. Place in a double boiler and stir frequently until the mixture melts and nearly all the sweetener dissolves.
3. Remove the bowl from the double boiler and let it cool for a few minutes.

4. Add eggs into the bowl of butter mixture, one at a time and stir well each time. Do not over beat. If the batter is too thick, add one more egg.
5. Stir in the almond flour. Whisk until well combined.
6. Pour batter into prepared baking dish.
7. Bake in a preheated oven 350° F for about 18 – 20 minutes or until it just sets in the middle. If you insert a toothpick, you should have a bit of the batter sticking to it.
8. Remove from the oven. Sprinkle flaky sea salt on top and let it cool on a wire rack completely.
9. Cut into 8 equal pieces and serve in bowls. Drizzle some macadamia milk over the brownies and serve.
10. Leftovers can be stored in an airtight container in the refrigerator for 6-7 days or frozen for 2 months.

Nutrition Info: Per Servings: Calories: 92.6 kcal, Fat: 7.9 g, Carbohydrates: 3.8 g, Protein: 1.5 g

Keto Pistachio Icebox Cake

Servings: 10

Cooking Time:20 Minutes

Ingredients:

- 1 cup finely chopped almonds (not ground almonds)
- ½ cup ground hazelnuts
- 4 oz butter, melted
- 2 cups heavy cream
- 1 ½ tsp Stevia/your preferred keto sweetener
- 3 egg yolks
- 1 cup chopped pistachios
- Few drops of green food coloring (optional)

Directions:

1. Grease a cake pan with butter and set aside
2. Combine the almonds, hazelnuts and melted butter in a bowl until they reach a wet sand consistency
3. Press the nut/butter mixture into the bottom of your prepared cake pan
4. Place ONE CUP of the cream, the sweetener and egg yolks into a saucepan and place over a medium heat
5. Whisk the cream/egg mixture as it heats and begins to thicken, remove from the heat and allow to cool
6. Whip the remaining cup of cream until thick and soft

7. Fold the whipped cream into the cooled cream/egg mixture until combined

8. Fold the pistachios and food coloring (if using) into the mixture and spoon into your nut-lined cake pan, smooth out the top

9. Cover the cake with plastic wrap and place into the freezer overnight

10. Slice and serve!

Nutrition Info: Calories: 406;Fat: 41 grams ;Protein: 7 grams ;Total carbs: 8 grams ;Net carbs: 5 grams

Sweet Blackberry Ice Cream

Servings: 8

Cooking Time: 30 Minutes

Ingredients:

- 1 egg yolks
- 1 cup blackberries
- ½ cup erythritol
- 1 ½ cup heavy whipping cream

Directions:

1. Add all ingredients to the bowl and blend until well combined.
2. Pour ice cream mixture into the ice cream maker and churn ice cream according to the machine instructions.
3. Serve and enjoy.

Nutrition Info: Per Servings: Net Carbs: 1.; Calories: 92; Total Fat: 9g; Saturated Fat: 5.4g Protein: 1.1g; Carbs: 2.4g; Fiber: 1g; Sugar: 0.9g; Fat 89% Protein 5% Carbs 6%

Coconut Butter Popsicle

Servings: 12

Cooking Time: 5 Minutes

Ingredients:

- 2 cans unsweetened coconut milk
- 1 tsp liquid stevia
- 12 cup peanut butter

Directions:

1. Add all ingredients into the blender and blend until smooth.
2. Pour mixture into the molds and place in the refrigerator for 3 hours or until set.
3. Serve and enjoy.

Nutrition Info: Per Servings: Net Carbs: 3.1g; Calories: 175 Total Fat: 17.; Saturated Fat: 10.7g Protein: 3.5g; Carbs: 3.7g; Fiber: 0.6g; Sugar: 2.6g; Fat 87% Protein 7% Carbs 6%

Frozen Coconut Blackberry Whip

Servings: 10

Cooking Time:15 Minutes

Ingredients:

- 1 ½ cups heavy cream
- 1 ½ cups full fat coconut cream
- 1 cup unsweetened toasted dried coconut
- 1 ½ tsp Stevia/your preferred keto sweetener
- 1 ½ cups blackberries

Directions:

1. Whip the cream until soft and fluffy
2. Whip the coconut cream until soft and fluffy (I find it easier to whip the cream and coconut cream separately)
3. Combine the whipped cream and coconut cream in a large bowl
4. Stir the toasted coconut, sweetener and blackberries into the whipped cream mixture
5. Spoon the mixture into an ice cream container or plastic container and place the lid on top
6. Place the container into the freezer and give it a vigorous stir every hour for the first five hours of freezing
7. Enjoy however you wish!

Nutrition Info: Calories: 2;Fat: 26 grams ;Protein: 2 grams ;Total carbs: 7 grams;Net carbs: 6 grams

Tangy Lime And Tequila Popsicles

Servings: 6

Cooking Time:10 Minutes

Ingredients:

- ½ cup fresh lime juice
- Juice of 2 lemons
- 1 tsp Stevia/your preferred keto sweetener
- 2 cups water
- 4 oz tequila

Directions:

1. Place all ingredients into a saucepan and bring to a simmer, remove from the heat and allow to cool completely
2. Stir the tequila into the mixture
3. Pour the mixture into popsicle molds and place into the freezer to freeze overnight
4. If you don't have popsicle molds, you could pour the mixture into a container and turn it into sorbet as opposed to individual popsicles

Nutrition Info: Calories: ;Fat: 0 gram;Protein: 0 gram;Total carbs: 3 grams ;Net carbs: 2 grams

Berries And Cream Popsicles

Servings: 4

Cooking Time: 0 Minute

Ingredients:

- 8 ounces of cream cheese softened
- 2 cups of heavy whipping cream
- 1 tablespoon of lemon juice
- 1/4 cup of sour cream
- 1 1/2 cups of fresh sliced strawberries
- 1 cup of fresh blueberries
- 3/4 cup of swerve

Directions:

1. Blend cream cheese with lemon juice, sour cream, and heavy cream in a food processor until smooth.
2. Add ½ cup blueberries, 1 cup strawberries, and sweetener.
3. Blender well until smooth.
4. Add remaining berries to the bottom of each popsicle mold.
5. Divide the cream cheese mixture into these molds.
6. Insert the ice cream stick into each mold.
7. Freeze them for about 4 hours or more.
8. Serve after removing from the molds.
9. Enjoy.

Nutrition Info: Per Servings: Calories 266 Total Fat 25.7 g Saturated Fat 1.2 g Cholesterol 41 mg Total Carbs 9.7 g Sugar 1.2 g Fiber 0.5 g Sodium 18 mg Potassium 78 mg Protein 2.6 g

Coconut

Servings: 14

Cooking Time: 40 Minutes

Ingredients:

- 1 large scoop protein powder, vanilla flavored
- 4 oz. dark chocolate chips, unsweetened
- 1 cup coconut, flaked
- 3/4 cup coconut oil, melted
- 1 1/2 cups macadamia nuts, raw

Directions:

1. Using an 8-inch pan, cover with baking paper or a non-stick mat.In a food blender set to high, blend the macadamia nuts and coconut oil until evenly mixed.
2. Combine the protein powder, chocolate chips, and coconut until mixed thoroughly.
3. Transfer the batter to the prepped pan and freeze for half an hour.
4. After it's set, slice into 1individual bars.
5. Thaw for 10 minutes before serving.
6. Tricks and Tips:
7. You can use other nuts in this recipe instead of macadamia. Experiment with cashews, walnuts, almonds or a mix.

Nutrition Info: 4 grams ;Net Carbs: 4 grams ;Fat: 20 grams ;Calories: 213

Classic Vanilla Ice Cream

Servings: 6

Cooking Time:20 Minutes

Ingredients:

- 3 cups heavy cream
- 2 Tbsp butter
- 1 tsp Stevia/your preferred keto sweetener
- 3 tsp vanilla extract
- ½ cup coconut oil

Directions:

1. Place TWO CUPS of cream into a saucepan with the butter, sweetener, vanilla and coconut oil, place over a medium heat
2. Allow the mixture to come to a simmer as you whisk. Remove from the heat and allow to cool
3. Beat the leftover one cup of cream until soft and thick
4. Fold the cooled cream/vanilla mixture into the whipped cream, being careful not to deflate the whipped cream too much
5. Pour the mixture into an ice cream container or plastic container, place the lid on top
6. Place the ice cream into the freezer and give it a stir every hour for the first five hours (if possible) to help the ice cream to become creamy and fluffy

7. Serve however you like!

Nutrition Info: Calories: 613;Fat: 66 grams ;Protein: 2 grams ;Total carbs: 4 grams;Net carbs: 4 grams

Avocado Sorbet

Servings: 5

Cooking Time: 10 Minutes

Ingredients:

- 2 avocados
- 2 cups unsweetened almond milk
- 2 tbsp fresh lime juice
- 34 cup Swerve
- 12 tsp sea salt

Directions:

1. Add all ingredients into the blender and blend until smooth.
2. Transfer blended mixture into the container and place in the refrigerator for 10 minutes.
3. After 5 minutes add sorbet mixture into the ice cream maker and churn according to the machine instructions.
4. Transfer into the air-tight container and place in the refrigerator for 1-2 hours.
5. Serve chilled and enjoy.

Nutrition Info: Per Servings: Net Carbs: 2.3g; Calories: 181; Total Fat: 17.1g; Saturated Fat: 3.4g Protein: 1.9g; Carbs: 8.1g; Fiber: 5.8g; Sugar: 0.4g; Fat 8 Protein 8% Carbs 6%

Berry Sorbet

Servings: 2

Cooking Time: 10 Minutes

Ingredients:

- 12 cup raspberries
- 12 cup strawberries
- 12 tsp liquid stevia
- 14 cup blackberries
- 1 tsp fresh lemon juice

Directions:

1. Add all ingredients into the blender and blend until smooth.
2. Pour into the container and place in the refrigerator for 3 hours.
3. Serve chilled and enjoy.

Nutrition Info: Per Servings: Net Carbs: 5g; Calories: 36; Total Fat: 1g; Saturated Fat: 0g Protein: 0.9g; Carbs: 8.2g; Fiber: 3.7g; Sugar: 4.1g; Fat 25% Protein 25% Carbs 50%

Blueberry Mint Popsicles

Servings: 2

Cooking Time: 20 Minutes

Ingredients:

- 1 can coconut milk
- 1/2 cup blueberries
- 1/2-ounce lime juice
- 2 tbsp mint leaves

Directions:

1. Let coconut milk simmer in a saucepan for 5 minutes with mint leaves.
2. Remove it from the heat then strain and allow it to cool.
3. Heat blueberries with lime juice in a saucepan over low, medium heat for 5 minutes.
4. Allow this berry compote to cool at room temperature.
5. Divide the coconut milk into the popsicle molds.
6. Freeze them for 30 minutes then remove the molds from the freezer.
7. Add berry compote to each mold and make swirls using a stick.
8. Insert ice cream sticks into the molds and freeze again for 2 hours or more.
9. Serve.

Nutrition Info: Per Servings: Calories 113 Total Fat 9 g Saturated Fat 0.2 g Cholesterol 1.7 mg Total Carbs 6.5 g Sugar 1.8 g Fiber 0.7 g Sodium 134 mg Potassium 123 mg Protein 7.5 g

Frozen Yogurt With Berries

Servings: 4

Cooking Time: 0 Minutes

Ingredients:

- 4 cups frozen blackberries
- 1 cup full-fat Greek yogurt
- 1 tablespoon lemon juice
- 1 teaspoon vanilla essence

Directions:

1. Beat everything in a food processor until smooth.
2. Transfer the yogurt mixture to a sealable bowl.
3. Place it in the freezer overnight.
4. Serve and enjoy.

Nutrition Info: Calories 113 ;Total Fat 9 g ;Saturated Fat 0.2 g ;Cholesterol 1.7 mg ;Sodium 134 mg ;Total Carbs 6.g ;Sugar 1.8 g ;Fiber 0.7 g ;Protein 7.5 g

Raspberry Lemon Popsicles

Servings: 2

Cooking Time: 0 Minute

Ingredients:

- 1 cup lemon juice
- 2 cups water
- 3 to 5 doonks of stevia
- ½ cup frozen raspberries, roughly chopped

Directions:

1. Divide the chopped berries into popsicle molds.
2. Mix lemon juice with stevia, and water in a bowl.
3. Divide this mixture into the popsicle molds and insert the ice cream sticks in it.
4. Freeze them for about hours or more.
5. Serve after removing from the molds.
6. Enjoy.

Nutrition Info: Per Servings: Calories 101 Total Fat 15.5 g Saturated Fat 4.5 g Cholesterol 12 mg Total Carbs 4.4 g Sugar 1.2 g Fiber 0.3 g Sodium 18 mg Potassium 128 mg Protein 4.8 g

Classic Citrus Custard

Servings: 4

Cooking Time: 10 Minutes

Ingredients:

- 2 ½ cups heavy whipping cream
- ½ tsp orange extract
- 2 tbsp fresh lime juice
- ¼ cup fresh lemon juice
- ½ cup Swerve
- Pinch of salt

Directions:

1. Boil heavy whipping cream and sweetener in a saucepan for 5-6 minutes. Stir continuously.
2. Remove saucepan from heat and add orange extract, lime juice, lemon juice, and salt and mix well.
3. Pour custard mixture into ramekins.
4. Place ramekins in refrigerator for 6 hours.
5. Serve chilled and enjoy.

Nutrition Info: Per Servings: Net Carbs: 2.7g; Calories: 2; Total Fat: 27.9g; Saturated Fat: 17.4g Protein: 1.7g; Carbs: 2.8g; Fiber: 0.1g; Sugar: 0.5g; Fat 94% Protein 2% Carbs 4%

Mango Yogurt Popsicles

Servings: 4

Cooking Time: 0 Minutes

Ingredients:

- 8 oz. frozen mango, diced
- 8 oz. frozen strawberries
- 1 cup Greek yogurt
- 2.5 teaspoons heavy whipping cream
- 1 teaspoon vanilla essence

Directions:

1. Beat everything in a food processor until it forms a smooth batter.
2. Divide this mixture into the popsicle molds.
3. Cover the molds and stick the popsicle sticks into the molds.
4. Place the popsicle in the freezer for hours.
5. Remove the popsicle from the molds.
6. Serve and enjoy.

Nutrition Info: Calories 19;Total Fat 19.2 g ;Saturated Fat 10.1 g ;Cholesterol 11 mg ;Sodium 78 mg ;Total Carbs 7.3 g ;Sugar 1.2 g ;Fiber 0.8 g ;Protein 4.2 g

Vanilla Yogurt

Servings: 4

Cooking Time: 15 Minutes

Ingredients:

- 1 vanilla pod (seeds)
- 1 teaspoon vanilla essence
- 1 13.5-ounce can full-fat coconut milk
- Erythritol, to taste
- 1/4 teaspoon salt
- 1/4 teaspoon xanthan gum
- 1 cup of coconut yogurt
- 2 teaspoons vanilla essence
- 1 tablespoon vodka

Directions:

1. Combine salt, coconut milk, erythritol and vanilla seeds in a saucepan.
2. Cook this milk mixture for 15 minutes on medium heat.
3. Stir in xanthan gum and whisk this mixture until frothy.
4. Strain it through a sieve in a to bowl then cover the mixture with a plastic wrap.
5. Place the bowl for 30 minutes in the refrigerator.

6. Add yogurt to a suitable bowl then add the refrigerator vanilla mixture and vanilla essence.

7. Mix well and churn it in an ice cream maker for 20 minutes.

8. Freeze it for 2 hours in the freezer then transfer it to a covered container.

9. Place it back in the refrigerator for 6 hours.

10. Serve and enjoy.

Nutrition Info: Calories 173 ;Total Fat 13 g ;Saturated Fat 10.1 g ;Cholesterol 12 mg ;Sodium 67 mg ;Total Carbs 7.5 g ;Sugar 1.2 g ;Fiber 0.6 g ;Protein 3.2 g

Cinnamon Ice Cream

Servings: 8

Cooking Time: 30 Minutes

Ingredients:

- 1 egg yolk
- ½ tsp vanilla
- 3 tsp cinnamon
- ¾ cup erythritol
- 2 cups heavy whipping cream
- Pinch of salt

Directions:

1. Add all ingredients to the mixing bowl and blend until well combined.
2. Pour ice cream mixture into the ice cream maker and churn ice cream according to the machine instructions.
3. Serve and enjoy.

Nutrition Info: Per Servings: Net Carbs: 1.1g; Calories: 113 Total Fat: 11.7g; Saturated Fat: 7.1g Protein: 1g; Carbs: 1.6g; Fiber: 0.5g; Sugar: 0.1g; Fat 93% Protein 3% Carbs

Cheesecake Vanilla Bites

Servings: 4

Cooking Time: 0 Minutes

Ingredients:

- 8 oz. cream cheese softened
- 1/2 cup butter softened
- 1/2 cup erythritol or sugar substitute
- 1/2 teaspoon vanilla essence

Directions:

1. Beat everything in a food processor until smooth.
2. Line a baking sheet with parchment paper.
3. Divide the mixture into a muffin tray.
4. Place the tray in the freezer for 1 hour.
5. Serve and enjoy.

Nutrition Info: Calories 147 ;Total Fat 11 g ;Saturated Fat 10.1 g ;Cholesterol 10 mg ;Sodium 91 mg ;Total Carbs 4.2 g ;Sugar 2 g ;Fiber 0.4 g ;Protein 3.2 g

Raspberry Yogurt

Servings: 6

Cooking Time: 10 Minutes

Ingredients:

- 2 cups plain yogurt
- 5 oz fresh raspberries
- ½ cup erythritol

Directions:

1. Add all ingredients into the blender and blend until smooth.
2. Transfer blended mixture in air-tight container and place in the refrigerator for 40 minutes.
3. Remove yogurt mixture from refrigerator and blend again until smooth.
4. Pour in container and place in the refrigerator for 30 minutes.
5. Serve and enjoy.

Nutrition Info: Per Servings: Net Carbs: 7g; Calories: 70 Total Fat: 1.9g; Saturated Fat: 0.8g Protein: 5.1g; Carbs: 8.5g; Fiber: 1.5g; Sugar: 8g; Fat 26% Protein 32% Carbs 42%

Protein Yogurt

Servings: 4

Cooking Time: 0 Minutes

Ingredients:

- 1 cup Greek yogurt full-fat
- 1 cup raspberries frozen
- 1 tablespoon coconut oil
- 1 tablespoon vanilla whey powder
- Stevia extract to taste
- 1 dash salt
- 1 tablespoon vodka optional - to taste

Directions:

1. Beat everything in a food processor until smooth.
2. Transfer the yogurt mixture to a sealable bowl.
3. Place it in the freezer for about 4 hours.
4. Serve and enjoy.

Nutrition Info: Calories 213 ;Total Fat 19 g ;Saturated Fat 12 g ;Cholesterol 13 mg ;Sodium 52 mg ;Total Carbs 5.5 g ;Sugar 1.3 g ;Fiber 0.5 g ;Protein 6.1 g

Chocolate Whips

Servings: 12

Cooking Time: 1 Hour 20 Minutes

Ingredients:

- 2 1/2 tbsp. Swerve sweetener, granulated
- 1/2 tsp. vanilla extract, sugar-free
- 3 tbsp. cocoa powder, unsweetened
- 8 tbsp. heavy whipping cream
- 1/8 tsp. salt

Directions:

1. Set a cookie sheet out and layer with baking paper.
2. In a stand mixer on high, whip the sweetener and vanilla extract for 60 seconds.
3. Blend the heavy whipping cream, salt and cocoa powder for additional minutes.
4. Scoop the whipped cream into a piping bag with a 1M nozzle.
5. Squeeze the contents on the prepared cookie sheet, creating individual swirls that look like ice cream on a cone.
6. Freeze for a minimum of 1 hour until firm and serve.
7. Tricks and Tips:

8. You can get creative with this recipe and try out other flavors. Simply substitute 1 teaspoon of flavored extract in place of the cocoa powder.

9. Don´t have a piping bag in your kitchen? You can alternatively use a gallon sized ziplock bag. Just add the whipped cream and cut one corner of the bottom to the size you prefer.

10. If you prefer soft serve ice cream, simply let the whips defrost for approximately minutes before serving.

11. These can be frozen for up to 2 months in a freezer safe container, but we do not think they will last that long!

Nutrition Info: 0 grams ;Net Carbs: 1.5 grams ;Fat: 8 grams ;Calories: 70

Raspberry Sorbet

Servings: 8

Cooking Time: 12 Hours And 5 Minutes

Ingredients:

- 1 ½ cups raspberries
- 1/4 cup erythritol sweetener
- 2 tablespoons gelatin
- 1 cup water

Directions:

1. Place all the ingredients in a blender and puree until smooth.
2. Pass the mixture through a strainer into a freezer bag, about 1 quart, and place in freezer for 4 hours until thickened, massaging every hour.
3. Then freeze for 6 to 8 hours or until completely firm.
4. When ready to serve, remove the bag from the freezer, thaw for 10 minutes at room temperature and then scoop into serving bowls.

Nutrition Info: Calories: 43 Cal, Carbs: g, Fat: 0 g, Protein: 1 g, Fiber: 3 g.

Pumpkin Ice Cream

Servings: 5

Cooking Time: 10 Minutes

Ingredients:

- 2 cups heavy whipping cream
- 1 ½ tsp liquid stevia
- 2 tsp pumpkin pie spice
- 1 tbsp vanilla
- ½ cup pumpkin puree

Directions:

1. Add all ingredients into the food processor and process until fluffy.
2. Transfer ice cream mixture in air-tight container and place in the refrigerator for 1 hour.
3. Remove ice cream mixture from refrigerator and whisk until smooth.
4. Again place in the refrigerator for 2 hours.
5. Serve chilled and enjoy.

Nutrition Info: Per Servings: Net Carbs: 3.3g; Calories: 184; Total Fat: 17.9g; Saturated Fat: 11.1g Protein: 1.3g; Carbs: 4.1g; Fiber: 0.8g; Sugar: 1.2g; Fat 88% Protein 4% Carbs 8%

Raspberry And Almond Froyo

Servings: 8

Cooking Time:10 Minutes

Ingredients:

- 1 cup heavy cream
- 2 cups full-fat Greek yogurt
- 1 ½ cups frozen raspberries
- ¾ cup slivered almonds, toasted
- 1 tsp Stevia/your preferred keto sweetener

Directions:

1. Whip the cream until it is soft, fluffy and thick but not buttery
2. Fold the yogurt, raspberries, almonds and sweetener into the cream until thoroughly combined
3. Transfer the yogurt mixture into an ice cream container or plastic container, place the lid on and pop it into the freezer
4. If you can, give the froyo a stir every hour for the first five hours. This will help the froyo to freeze into a thick, creamy, fluffy texture
5. Serve and enjoy!

Nutrition Info: Calories: 2;Fat: 23 grams ;Protein: 6 grams ;Total carbs: 9 grams ;Net carbs: 7 grams

Tiramisu Ice Bombs

Servings: 12

Cooking Time: 3 Hours And 15 Minutes

Ingredients:

- For the Ice Bombs:
- 1/4 cup erythritol sweetener
- 2 teaspoons rum extract, unsweetened
- 1/4 cup strong brewed coffee, chilled
- 1 1/4 cups coconut milk, full-fat and unsweetened
- For the Coating:
- 1 ¼ tablespoon chocolate
- 1 tablespoon cacao butter

Directions:

1. Place all the ingredients for ice bombs in a food processor and pulse at high speed for to 2 minutes or until smooth and creamy.
2. Divide the mixture evenly between 1candy molds or round cake mold and freeze for 2 to 3 hours or until set and firm.
3. When ready to serve, place chocolate and cacao butter in a heatproof bowl and microwave for 45 seconds or more until melted and stir well.

4. Pierce each frozen ice bomb with a toothpick and coat with melted chocolate completely and place on a parchment lined a baking tray.

5. Place tray into the freezer for 1minutes or more until harden.

6. Serve straight away or store in plastic bag in the freezer.

Nutrition Info: Calories: 25 Cal, Carbs: 0.9 g, Fat: 2.3 g, Protein: 0.2 g, Fiber: 0.2 g.

Blueberry Almond Ice Cream Pops

Servings: 8

Cooking Time:15 Minutes

Ingredients:

- 3 cups heavy cream
- 3 egg yolks
- 1 ½ tsp Stevia/your preferred keto sweetener
- Few drops of almond essence
- ¾ cup chopped almonds, toasted
- 1 cup fresh blueberries

Directions:

1. Place TWO CUPS of the cream, the egg yolks, sweetener and almond essence into a saucepan and whisk to combine
2. Place the saucepan over a medium heat and keep whisking as the mixture heats and begins to thicken
3. Take the saucepan off the heat and set aside to cool
4. Whip the remaining cup of cream until soft and fluffy
5. Gently stir together the cooled egg yolk/cream mixture and whipped cream
6. Fold the chopped almonds and blueberries into the mixture
7. Spoon the mixture into your popsicle molds and pop into the freezer to freeze overnight

8. Before serving, leave the popsicle molds out at room temperature for a few minutes before sliding the ice creams out and passing around to eager guests!

Nutrition Info: Calories: 314;Fat: 31 grams ;Protein: 4 grams ;Total carbs: 6 grams;Net carbs: 5 grams

Peanut Butter Ice Cream Cupcakes

Servings: 8

Cooking Time:20 Minutes

Ingredients:

- 2 cups heavy cream
- 1 tsp Stevia/your preferred keto sweetener
- 4 Tbsp peanut butter (any kind, as long as it's natural and unsweetened)
- 3 egg yolks
- Frosting:
- 5 oz plain, full-fat cream cheese
- ½ cup heavy cream
- ½ tsp Stevia/your preferred keto sweetener

Directions:

1. Line 8 muffin holes in a muffin pan with cupcake cases and set aside
2. Place ONE CUP of the cream into a saucepan with the stevia and peanut butter, bring to a gentle simmer then take off the heat
3. Spoon a little of the hot cream mixture into the egg yolks and quickly whisk
4. Transfer the egg yolk mixture into the saucepan of cream mixture and place back onto a low heat, stirring as it thickens, set aside to cool

5. Whip the remaining one cup of cream until soft and fluffy
6. Fold the whipped cream into the cream/peanut butter mixture until combined
7. Spoon the mixture into the cupcake cases and put in the freezer as you make the frosting
8. To make the frosting: beat together the cream cheese, cream and sweetener until thick and smooth
9. Spoon the cream cheese mixture over the peanut butter cupcakes and pop back into the freezer
10. Eat the cupcakes when they're frozen but not totally hard (leaving them out for minutes at room temperature helps)

Nutrition Info: Calories: 379;Fat: 38 grams ;Protein: 5 grams ;Total carbs: 6 grams ;Net carbs: 5 grams

Mixed Berry Yogurt

Servings: 6

Cooking Time: 10 Minutes

Ingredients:

- 2 tbsp erythritol
- ½ lemon juice
- 1 tsp vanilla
- 1 cup coconut cream
- 1 cup mixed berries

Directions:

1. In a bowl, mix together coconut cream, sweetener, lemon juice, and vanilla and place in the refrigerator for 30 minutes.
2. Add berries and frozen coconut cream mixture into the blender and blend until smooth.
3. Transfer blended mixture in container and place in the refrigerator for 1-2 hours.
4. Serve and enjoy.

Nutrition Info: Per Servings: Net Carbs: 3.; Calories: 108; Total Fat: 9.7g; Saturated Fat: 8.5g Protein: 1.1g; Carbs: 5.2g; Fiber: 1.7g; Sugar: 3.2g; Fat 82% Protein 5% Carbs 13%

Lemon Cheese Ice Cream

Servings: 4

Cooking Time: 15 Minutes

Ingredients:

- 1 medium lemon, wash, peeled and remove seeds
- 3 tbsp swerve
- 1 cup of sparkling water
- 14 oz mascarpone cheese
- Pinch of sea salt

Directions:

1. Add all ingredients into the blender and blend until smooth and creamy.
2. Pour into the container and place in the refrigerator for hours.
3. Serve chilled and enjoy.

Nutrition Info: Per Servings: Net Carbs: 5.5g; Calories: 181; Total Fat: 12.9g; Saturated Fat: 8.2g Protein: 11.3g; Carbs: 5.9g; Fiber: 0.; Sugar: 0.6g; Fat 64% Protein 24% Carbs 12%

Chocolate-covered Macadamia Nut Fat Bombs

Servings: 4

Cooking Time: 40 Minutes

Ingredients:

- 1 ½ ounce macadamia nuts halves
- ¼ cup chocolate chips, stevia-sweetened
- 1/8 teaspoon sea salt and more as needed
- 1 tablespoon avocado oil

Directions:

1. Place chocolate chips in a heatproof bowl and microwave for 50 to 60 seconds or until melted.
2. Stir chocolate, and then stir in salt and oil until blended.
3. Take 8 mini muffin cups, place three nuts into each cup and then evenly spoon prepared chocolate mixture, covering nuts completely.
4. Sprinkle with more salt and chill in the freezer for 30 minutes or more until solid.
5. Serve straightaway or store in a plastic bag into the freezer.

Nutrition Info: Calories: 1 Cal, Carbs: 4 g, Fat: 16 g, Protein: 2 g, Fiber: 2 g.

Perfect Mint Ice Cream

Servings: 8

Cooking Time: 45 Minutes

Ingredients:

- 1 egg yolk
- ¼ tsp peppermint extract
- ½ cup erythritol
- 1 ½ cups heavy whipping cream

Directions:

1. Add all ingredients to the bowl and blend until well combined.
2. Pour ice cream mixture into the ice cream maker and churn ice cream according to the machine instructions.
3. Serve and enjoy.

Nutrition Info: Per Servings: Net Carbs: 0.7g; Calories: 85; Total Fat: 8.9g; Saturated Fat: 5. Protein: 0.8g; Carbs: 0.7g; Fiber: 0g; Sugar: 0.1g; Fat 94% Protein 3% Carbs 3%

Peanut Butter Ice Cream

Servings: 8

Cooking Time: 45 Minutes

Ingredients:

- 2 tbsp unsweetened cocoa powder
- 2 egg yolks
- ½ cup erythritol
- ½ cup peanut butter
- 2 cups heavy whipping cream

Directions:

1. In a large bowl, whisk together 2 tablespoons of warm water and cocoa powder.
2. Add remaining ingredients to the bowl and blend using blender until well combined.
3. Pour ice cream mixture into the ice cream maker and churn ice cream according to the machine instructions.
4. Serve and enjoy.

Nutrition Info: Per Servings: Net Carbs: 3.; Calories: 215; Total Fat: 20.5g; Saturated Fat: 9.1g Protein: 5.6g; Carbs: 4.9g; Fiber: 1.4g; Sugar: 1.6g; Fat 84% Protein 10% Carbs 6%

Vanilla Panna Cotta

Servings: 4

Cooking Time: 3 Hours And 15 Minutes

Ingredients:

- 2 tablespoons pomegranate seeds
- 1 teaspoon erythritol sweetener
- 2 teaspoons gelatin
- 1 tablespoon vanilla extract, unsweetened
- 2 cups heavy whipping cream, full-fat
- Water as needed

Directions:

1. Place gelatin in a small bowl and stir in small amount of water according to instructions on the pack, or tablespoon water for 1 teaspoon of gelatin and set aside until bloom.

2. In the meantime, place a saucepan over medium heat, add sweetener, vanilla, and cream and bring to boil.

3. Then lower heat to medium-low level and simmer mixture for to 4 minutes or until mixture begins to thicken.

4. Remove pan from heat, stir in gelatin until dissolved completely and then evenly divide between ramekins.

5. Cool ramekins at room temperature, then cover with plastic wrap and chill in the refrigerator for 2 to 3 hours.

6. When ready to serve, thaw pannacotta at room temperature, then top with pomegranate seeds and serve.

Nutrition Info: Calories: 422 Cal, Carbs: 4 g, Fat: 43 g, Protein: 4 g, Fiber: 0 g.

Frozen Yogurt

Servings: 8

Cooking Time: 1 Hour

Ingredients:

- 3 cups plain yogurt, full fat and chilled
- 1 tbsp. MCT oil
- 2 tsp. vanilla extract, sugar-free
- 1 tbsp. lemon juice
- 4 tbsp. monk fruit sweetener, confectioner
- 8 tsp. blueberry syrup, sugar-free (optional)

Directions:

1. In a food blender set on medium, blend the lemon juice, MCT oil, and sweetener for 2 minutes until incorporated.
2. Add the yogurt and vanilla extract and stir in with a rubber scraper.
3. Place the bowl in the freezer for half an hour.
4. Once set, top with the blueberry syrup, if you prefer, and serve.
5. Tricks and Tips:
6. This recipe is for soft serve yogurt. If you would like it to be harder, leave in the freezer for hours before serving.

Nutrition Info: 3 grams ;Net Carbs: 2.grams ;Fat: 11 grams ;Calories: 122

Lightning Source UK Ltd.
Milton Keynes UK
UKHW021302100521
383455UK00005B/69